Remember!
Re-act!
J. C. White

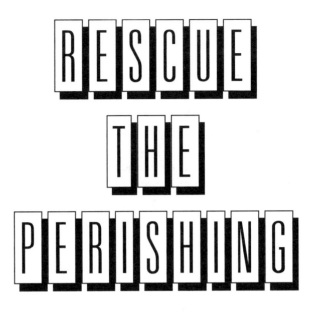

RESCUE THE PERISHING

JEANNE C. WHITE

American Literary Press, Inc.
Five Star Special Edition
Baltimore, Maryland

RESCUE THE PERISHING

Library of Congress
Cataloging in Publication Data
ISBN 1-56167-730-2

Library of Congress Card Catalog Number:
2001119897

Published by

American Literary Press, Inc.
Five Star Special Edition
8019 Belair Road, Suite 10
Baltimore, Maryland 21236

Manufactured in the United States of America

RESCUE THE PERISHING is dedicated to a little girl, who entered my life in 1993, and who has changed it forever; to my devoted husband, Mac, my friend, whose heart was also captured by this little girl, and who has unselfishly embraced the desire to rescue at least one child; and my daughter, Stephanie, who has always understood the cause of her mother's devotion to children, and to my granddaughter, Camille. My story is true, but the names have been changed and details added for effect.

SOMEBODY'S CHILD

Somebody's child, stricken from birth,
With full blown AIDS, a scourge on earth.
With crippled legs, she could not stand,
Yet trusted all and gave me her hand.

Somebody's child stole my heart,
A very great presence 'til death us did part.
When three years old, she lost her fight.
I held her hand through the approaching night.

Somebody's child lies far away,
In an unmarked grave, bleak and gray.
Gone! Forgotten! No honor! No fame!
Because of her, I'm not the same.

Introduction

"Genesis"

"Some men are born great; some men achieve greatness, and some have greatness thrust upon them."

William Shakespeare

The last clause of this quotation applies to a little girl with doelike eyes, who entered my life in the spring of 1993, and who, as a result of this book, will be a catalyst for change, now, and in years to come. Let me backtrack a little to my life prior to meeting one who will be known as Mylia. I was basking in retirement from a career of teaching English in the Baltimore City Public Schools. Part of my time was spent as a volunteer/substitute at the Barton School. As an intellect and a socially conscious person, I had kept abreast of current events including the AIDS epidemic, but I had not been touched personally by the disease. I believed that AIDS happened to "other" people, and resulted from "chosen" lifestyles. Aside from reading a few articles in magazines and watching stories on television, I had no ready frame of reference for the havoc and devastation that this disease wrecks upon its victim, and their families.

Mylia, not only changed my attitude, but she changed the focus and course of my life, and gave me a "mission." There was an instant bonding with this little one, who in addition to being HIV positive, had cerebral palsy, and was a "ward of the state." In no time, I began to envision myself in the role of her guardian. Her name began to come up daily at the dinner table.

The more I interacted with Mylia, the more I loved her; the more I thirsted for knowledge about AIDS, the more I realized that in cloaking victims in shrouds of confidentiality, we have done them a great injustice; the more I questioned the suitability of the foster homes in which Mylia had been placed, the more I sought to understand how child welfare agencies operate. Finally, in recognition of Mylia's worth and value as a human being, and the many others like her, who deserve a stable, loving, and happy home, my husband and I decided to work our way through the "system" in hopes of rescuing one child.

Application

Mylia, and others like her, will "have greatness thrust upon them," and this book will have achieved its purpose, if after reading it, the following actions result:

1. One person believes that AIDS cannot be acquired through loving and taking care of a victim.
2. One person rescues a child from an institution or hospital, and provides a quality life for this child, until the child is united with his or her family, or until he or she dies, thus eliminating the "many homes" syndrome that many children in foster care experience.
3. One retired couple decides to become foster parents to one child who is HIV positive.
4. One person decides to stop using drugs, engaging in "unsafe" sex, etc. in order to prevent a child from being born with AIDS.
5. One church, fraternity, sorority, club, etc., adopts the family caring for a child with AIDS, and facilitates outings, friendship, etc.
6. One "pro-life" supporter decides to substitute time, money, and support to a child stricken with AIDS, in place of signs and pickets.
7. One child welfare organization manages to eliminate the "red tape," especially when a couple, have not only met all the steps in the licensing process, but have specified a preference for one with AIDS.
8. The "public" actively supports an increase in funding for research.
9. No child dies alone, shunned, or forgotten, because no adult cared enough to be there until the "end."

CONTENTS

Chapter 1

The Barton School

It is 8:00 a.m., a weekday, and an early morning haze is beginning to lift on Barton Avenue in southwest Baltimore. It will be warm and sunny today, but the haze that surrounds the school will remain, partly due to the massive awning on the front of the school, and because the sun is either blocked by the tall buildings that surround the school, or by the half-century-old trees that make up a great portion of the landscape.

The Barton School a huge, impressive, weather-beaten structure that, with its tranquil grounds, occupies about one city block. Its facade on Barton Avenue, faces the expansive campus of Caldor State College. The school also abuts Wayne Avenue and Wellwood Avenue, both of which feature single family porch front homes, fronted with neatly manicured lawns. To the south of the school, too close for comfort, lies a section of South Avenue that bears no resemblance to its former "glory" days. Its decaying houses accent what occurs in the city when once privately owned houses become rentals and apartments.

The school opened for occupancy in 1900 to perpetuate the memory of a renowned therapist. Its original purpose was to serve physically handicapped white children, but the current population of about 160 children encompasses children of all races.

The school, which includes three stories, is situated on an eight acre site, 770 x 335 feet, with the actual building taking up

300 x 250 feet. In stark contrast to the modern streamlined buildings on the campus of the college and the homes in the two adjacent neighborhoods, the school brings to mind a Gothic structure and is both majestic and haunting.

Inside, the presence of wheel chairs in all shapes, sizes, and colors lined up neatly in the foyer suggest immediately that this is not the usual public school. Immaculate, shiny floors in the corridors and rooms, up-to-date creative bulletin boards, displays, showcases, and learning nooks, all echo the vital lesson of acceptance that the school imparts. Just outside of the main office, on a wall beneath huge oil paintings of former administrators, one can read the eloquent mission of the school:

The mission is to provide appropriate academic and therapeutic programs for children with handicapping conditions from birth to 18 years of age by facilitating their physical, academic, social, and emotional growth in all developmental areas through various activities involving school, family, and community in order to prepare them to live productively.

The execution of this mission is accomplished by an army of special people, who because of their love and devotion, can see beyond the physical handicap of each child, beyond each seemingly impossibility, and into each soul and the realm of possibility. The army includes the administrators, a teacher for each class, an assistant for each class, occupational and physical therapists, music, etc., nurses, cafeteria personnel, custodians, and volunteers. A student- teacher ratio of 4 to 1 enables each student to be nurtured, instructed, and challenged.

Chapter 2

Staff and Students

Articulating the day today operational activities is a Herculean task that seems to be accomplished effortlessly by the principal. Though miles from resembling a "drill sergeant," she has an aura surrounding her that affirms her commitment to "getting the job done, getting it done well, and getting it done as a team effort."

She is warm and charismatic, and she packs a lot of persuasiveness in her 5 feet 4 inch pleasingly plump frame. Her neatly coiffed business hair style is speckled with gray; her youthful face belies her age, but blends in perfectly with her physical agility and high energy level.

It is 8: 30 a.m., and all under her management, the staff is moving into place on both Barton and Wayne Avenues. At both sites, in assembly line precision, twenty-two "cheese" busses in all will be unloaded and all of the passengers delivered safely to their classrooms.

By 8:45, the halls bustle with activity. An air of happiness and expectation pervades as the students move "en masse." Some walk with awkward, lunging gaits, holding tightly to walkers and canes; others steer their manual or electric chairs themselves, fending off any offers of assistance. The infants and toddlers, who have been unstrapped from the car seats in which they have sat, in some instances for over an hour, are next secured in wheelchairs through a complicated looking assortment of belts and straps. Each of the students has brought a bookbag that contains such items as books, and pencils, as well as pampers, extra clothing, eyeglasses, hearing aids, splints, and in some cases, computers.

The trained eye can identify those with Downs Syndrome, spina bifida, and cerebral palsy. Some students have multiple impairments, but in spite of everything, they come expecting to have a great day. One of my friends remarked, not at all unkindly, she wouldn't be able to work at a school such as Barton because it would depress her. I responded by citing the "special" nature of the staff at the school. These men and women are able to look beyond the disability a student has to envision where he or she is today, and where through love and encouragement, etc., he or she can be in the future. It would do a chronic complainer much good to spend just one day in the company of these students. I dare to believe that this person would end up so in awe of their tenacity and strength that ordinary complaints would no longer matter.

By 9:00 a.m., all of the student are in their rooms. The halls that bustled fifteen minutes ago are now quiet. The two creaky elevators that delivered younger children to the ground floor are now still, but only until 2:00 p.m. Then the entire process will be repeated in reverse. For now, all eyes and hearts are tuned up for another wonderful day.

Chapter 3

In the Company of an Angel

Into this setting, in April of 1993, comes a new enrollee in the "Infant and Toddler" program. As she is unstrapped from her car seat, brought into the school, and transferred to a wheelchair, she holds tightly to the adults with an innocent trust; yet there is fear and apprehension in her doelike eyes. Her name is Mylia, and she is a pretty, twenty-two pound, twenty-eight month old Afro-American, who looks and acts much younger than her age. Her fragility is accented by her outfit, lovingly assembled, as I would later learn, by her first "foster mom." She is wearing a pale pink cotton dress, edged with lace, white shoes and socks. A wisp of fine, curly hair escapes from her matching bonnet. A greeting from the staff member who is operating the elevator causes Mylia to smile, one of those smiles that will jolt one's soul, and that will become her dearest characteristic, particularly in view of the neglect that she has experienced, and the pain she has felt, and will continue to feel because of her health problems. The fact that she doesn't utter a sound is not unusual for one so young in a new setting, but, later on, will be cited as one of the signs of neglect.

When the elevator stops at the ground floor, Mylia comes face to face with her teacher, Miss Lacy Wilcox, who will, like Anne Sullivan did for Helen Keller, "open up the world" for her. The fear and apprehension vanish from her eyes, and although it is not known at the moment, the love between these two will be so strong, that a year later, when Mylia is still calling all females "Mama," she will excitedly call "Lacy" each day as she nears her classroom. What makes Miss, Lacy so special? First, blond hair, that falls in cascades around her shoulders, gives Mylia something to grasp. Then Miss Lacy is a nurturer and has a talent for "mothering" despite the fact that she has no children of her own. Youthful and in her early thirties, Miss Lacy conveys a spontaneity and enthusiasm that is contagious. At about 5 feet 2 inches tall and at about 140 pounds, she does not frighten toddlers as some adults do. Her soft slow manner of speaking soothes Mylia, and in less than thirty minutes in her well appointed, bright, curiosity-provoking room, Mylia is contentedly snacking on orange juice and "Fruit Loops" with seven other toddlers. During "circle time," as Miss Lacy leads an "action" song about a school bus, Mylia watches and imitates Miss Lacy, and it is apparent immediately, that Miss Lacy will be the "one" to unlock Mylia's intellect and help her to catch up with her peers.

By the time that I meet Mylia, she has staked out her own niche in Miss Lacy's heart and in the class. Cerebral palsy has prevented her from standing and walking on her own, but does not stop her from moving around the room. She scoots forward, sort of thrusting her body in the direction that she wants to go. She is beginning to speak, not in phrases and sentences, but through simple words and gestures. A large cardboard box that has been made into a house has become her favorite spot. Not only is Mylia socializing with her classmates, but she is kind and affectionate towards them. Miss Lacy has made it a practice of singing to Mylia while she changes her, and as a result, she knows "The Barney Song."

My love for this little one is frightening. I am becoming, I fear, obsessed. My heart aches when I learn that she is HIV positive, and is a "ward of the state" as a result of parental neglect. Now it is clear why silent panic engulfs her, if for some reason, Miss Lacy has to leave the room, and why at "naptime," she will not close her eyes. Her bottle is her "security blanket," and even though she eats next to nothing, she lusts for her bottle, continuing to grip it long after the milk is gone.

Even though I have a Masters in special education that qualifies me to work with older children, I find myself, because of Mylia, electing to spend more and more of my time with the infants and toddlers. Because of rusty parenting skills and no experience with pampers (Cloth diapers were the vogue in my day.), it takes me fifteen minutes initially to change her. All of the little ones in the class seem so fragile, that despite my practical nurse's training, I fear that I might hurt them if I rush.

When Miss Lacy's assistant quits, I literally jump at the chance to take her place until another assistant is hired. Doing so will enable me to spend much time with Miss Lacy, a person of such character and integrity that we have progressed, from respecting each other as professionals, to being friends, as well as enabling me to daily interact with Mylia. Miss Lacy reminds me again of the need to take "universal precautions" and of the need to protect Mylia's confidential medical history. She gives me the opportunity to share any personal fears or concerns. I have none, my stance being that I can be more of a threat to the child, than she is to me, because of the weakness of her immune system.

I do admit to Miss Lacy that I am emotionally involved. I articulate feelings of rage, helplessness, and frustration that this beautiful child, with an iron will to survive, will, through no fault of her own, face a shortened life, numerous infections, etc., with no family of her own. It doesn't surprise me that Miss Lacy feels these emotions also.

Daily encounters with the realities of pediatric AIDS, strengthen my resolve to do all in my power to make Mylia feel loved, secure, and comfortable. I eat a more balanced diet, increase my intake of vitamin C, get more rest, and even avoid people with colds to keep from posing a risk to her or having to miss a day. I learn to recognize signs of the illness such as thrush on the tongue, low grade fever, coughs, ear and throat infections, nose bleeds, diarrhea, etc.

Each day with Miss Lacy is filled with creative activities which enable Mylia to blossom. Her vocabulary is increasing; she is crawling instead of scooting, and she is singing lots of songs in tune. She looks forward to music resource class. It is in this class that the teacher and I recognize almost simultaneously, that Mylia has an "ear" for music. While changing her, I teach her "Do You Know The Muffin Man?" which she learns quickly, and sings for Miss Lacy in a soft, weak voice.

There are many days when Mylia does not feel well. Yet she "wills" herself to participate in every activity. I wish I could capture and freeze on film some of the special moments. By June 1993, my husband, Mac, not only knows, by name, all of the children in Miss Lacy's class, but he knows that one of them has captured my heart. This is even more apparent when I, who had always anticipated and looked forward to summers off, tell him that, since the infants and toddlers will continue in school for the summer, I will volunteer two days each week.

The Barton School is an old building, and it lacks many of the modern amenities such as central conditioning and air conditioning units. Temperatures can soar to the point of being unbearable. On days I spend with Mylia, I am oblivious to the heat. In light of her problems, life for me is a "crystal stair."

School opens in the fall of 1993, and a new assistant has been hired for Miss Lacy, I am both jealous and relieved. The jealousy surfaces when I realize that someone else will receive the love that Mylia generously gives; the relief surfaces when I realize that I won't have to come on a daily basis. I feel I need to wean myself from her so that she isn't constantly in my thoughts. However, major upheavals in her life impact adversely upon her and provide a target for the rage that I have been feeling. For a reason unknown to her teacher and me, Mylia is moved to a different foster home. She has been moved from a home in which there are no other children, to one in which the couple have small children of their own; she works at night, and he works in the day. Anger boils up and threatens to engulf me, but I smother it until I arrive at home. Mac and I wonder how the child welfare agents can rationalize such a placement for one with so many special needs. No matter how good the intentions of the foster family, we know that day-to-day life with Mylia will be extremely time consuming. There is no doubt in our minds that relocating Mylia will trigger separation anxiety stresses that will manifest in a deterioration of her health.

Until now, I have merely fantasized about becoming Mylia's guardian, but I begin to openly explore the feasibility of the idea with Mac. Sight unseen, he has grown to love this little angel just from hearing about her at dinnertime. For retirees, ages 54 and 64 respectively, just the thought of providing twenty-four hour care to a toddler is mind-blowing, not to mention alone one with Mylia's needs. But like me, he feels that Mylia needs and deserves more than being bounced from one place to another.

Back at school, I observe Mylia more closely. Each day she sports new clothes and seems to be receiving good care. I search her little face for signs of anxiety, but there are none. Each day I discuss her adjustment with Mac. Both of us want and need to feel "all is well" for her sake and for ours, thereby eliminating the impetus to act on our thoughts.

Two weeks later, on a Friday afternoon, Mylia does not ride home on the bus, but is picked up by someone unknown to me, and delivered to another foster home. I see how tightly she holds on to the one who has come for her, and I can imagine and feel her panic when she is left later the same day, abandoned, at the mercy of strangers, cast off, as if she is incapable of remembering faces and places.

This time the tears come, and I am not ashamed. The entire weekend passes with neither one of us able to get Mylia out of our minds. We wonder, if we had acted sooner on our thoughts, and had begun the licensing procedure, would we have her now.

We decide to self-educate ourselves about AIDS, and most importantly, to set in motion the process of becoming foster parents, so that if Mylia's current placement does not workout, we can be considered.

The self-education part is easiest to effect. Although there are not enough materials available, we explore every avenue. We voraciously devour every bit of information from pamphlets, medical journals, fiction and nonfiction, in our quest to be as knowledgeable as possible. We undergo a "spiritual baptism" from reading *And the Band Played On* by Randy Shilts and *No Time To Wait* by Nick Siano.

Setting in motion the process of becoming foster parents proves harder. Since there are many "child welfare organizations," all of which differ in training/licensing polices, support services, etc., Mac and I decide to hope for the best for Mylia in her new foster home, and to give ourselves more time to find out about and assess the various agencies.

Meanwhile, from my vantage point, Mylia seems to be adjusting to her home. She comes to school in "mint" condition, and as before, she sports new outfits. Her foster parents are very religious and, along with Mylia, have another foster child. Again, I question their ability to understand all that is entailed in meeting Mylia's needs. I do not underestimate the power of prayer, but in Mylia's case, prayer needs to be combined with action in order to detect signs of, and to avert "crisis."

The occurrence of more colds and infections suggests a deterioration of her health, but Mylia continues to flash her "million dollar smile." Several times recently, she has had a fever and has been sent home. She has had more frequent ear and throat infections. Daily she now arrives with thick clogged particles in her nose. Careful and strategic probing is necessary in order to avert a nose bleed. She has a chronic cough, and often has irritations under her nose and on her lips. I believe she is getting good care, but I think she grieves for the familiar faces she has known, the favorite toys she has played with, and the pets that have vanished.

As she does with all her little ones, Miss Lacy calls her home when Mylia doesn't "show" one Friday in November 1993. She learns that "my baby," as I now refer to her, is in Union Hospital. A lump rises in my throat, a lump that stays there until the following Monday. The day after I learn of her hospitalization, a most dreary and chilly Saturday, Mac and I set off for the hospital.

Finding a place to park in the general vicinity proves difficult, for this teaching hospital's buildings, labs, pharmacy, library, etc., form a "city" in itself, but we persevere and find a spot two blocks away from the main entrance. It doesn't matter that we are drenched as we approach the information desk, nor that we have no idea how to find Mylia in this monstrous place. Mac elects to remain in the first floor lounge, and I, after a few incorrect turns, locate "Pediatrics."

I spot Mylia, sitting in a high chair directly across from the nurse's station. Her tiny frail body appears to be dwarfed by the chair even though it is designed for a little child. She is dressed in an oversized shirt, and she is holding a piece of a puzzle. Upon hearing her name, she looks in my direction, and I believe, at that moment, that death is imminent. Her eyes are dull and sunk back into her head; there is a reddish purple swelling under each eye, and there are signs of a recent nosebleed. Because she is connected to an IV pole, I make no attempt to pick her up. I am terrified by the way that she looks, and have the unreasonable fear, that if I disturb her in any way she'll die. My visit is brief, but long enough for me to wonder why, not one person, asks who I am, or what my relationship to Mylia is. I am on an emotional "roller coaster" ride and I need to blame someone or something. If no one cares enough to monitor Mylia's visitors, what's to stop her "birth" mother from appearing, possibly upsetting her, or far worse, kidnapping her?

Once back on the main floor, I nearly collide with Mac, who has been scanning the host of people moving in all directions, so as not to lose me. He reads my face and asks nothing. He reads my fears, and they become his also. When we return the next day, Mylia is beginning to "bounce" back, something that will recur with subsequent bouts of illness. Her body is tolerating the antibiotics being administered to attack pneumonia, and she no longer has a fever.

My emotions are still controlling my thoughts, and I convince myself, that because Mylia is a "foster child," she will not get the best of care. I appoint myself as her "advocate," and without coercion, elicit Mac's support. We vow to come to the hospital whenever Mylia is a patient. Mac will drop me off at 9:00 a.m. and return at 3:00 p.m. If she is very ill, I will just rock her and play soft music. If she's better, we will sing familiar songs, color and go to the "playroom."

Unfortunately, Mylia continues to have health problems. Most people recover from colds, sore throats, and viruses during the season of winter, but she lacks the resistance to fight off these ailments. We find ourselves at the hospital more regularly. This is actually good because I see proof that my prior opinions of the staff towards Mylia are totally irrational.

As I interact more with the staff, it is clear that Mylia has captured many of their hearts also. They recognize her and remember her name. No one seems afraid to touch her, play with her, etc. Everyone wants to see her smile. The nurses and doctors grow used to seeing me. They answer my questions honestly, and in no way, condescendingly. When the nurses realize that I know how to care for Mylia's hygiene, and that I want to do it, they allow me to proceed. It is important to me that they view me, not as a "troublemaker," "busybody," or "do-gooder," but as Mylia's friend, "fairy godmother," and advocate.

Whatever I learn from the staff, I pass on to her foster dad when he comes on his lunch break. I never run into her foster mom, but it seems that she comes in the evening. "Jealousy" pops its head up again. I want to be Mylia's mother. There is a bed in her well-planned room, a spacious bathroom, and the availability of balanced meals at affordable prices. There is no excuse for her isolation! Who is there when she has a bad dream? Hurts? Cries? I want to be there.

It is good that Mylia is being served at the Union Hospital, for as a teaching hospital, it offers many amenities for patients, staff, etc. Its pediatric facility is vast and equipped with "state of the art" equipment. I am pleasantly surprised to discover that it has a clinic devoted to pediatric AIDS patients. In this respect, Mylia is blessed.

JEANNE C. WHITE

Chapter 4

Moments To Remember

The winter of 1993 holds many precious memories that overshadow the unpleasant ones. An unknown author wrote in "The Measure Of A Man" these words:

Not—how did he die? but—how did he live?
Not—what did he gain? but—what did he give?
These are the units to measure the worth
Of a man, as a man, regardless of birth.

Because Mylia gives so much just by "being," the poet's advice to all, "to live in the present," is not taken lightly.

The best memory that Mac has is of the day when she "hooks" him. On this day, Mylia is back in the hospital, recovering from another crisis. Instead of just dropping me off as usual, he decides to accompany me. Fortunately, the gift shop opens promptly at 9:00 a.m., and he finds the perfect balloon. Now, on the previous day, Mylia had been too weak to even sit up with assistance, but on this day, when she sees the balloon, she laughs and pulls her little crippled leg into a half-standing position. By some miracle, she is able to touch the balloon before her legs give out. She hasn't been prepared for the day, so I proceed to give her a "bed bath." Suddenly, with eyes only for Mac, in a weak soft voice, she sings "The Barney Song." There are tears in his eyes, and I know that, like me, Mac sees the value and purpose of this child, and he will never be the same.

Another memory is of her taking medicine. Mylia accepts her dosages of Valium and AZT in the same manner as another child accepts cookies. It is quite unsettling to see one so young, so stoic.

My fondest memory is of her third birthday which occurs the day after my 55th, making it impossible for me to ever forget. It is customary for the children in Miss Lacy's class to have parties at school. We decide to supplement the items that her foster mom promises to send and also to attend the party, as the mothers of the other children usually do. Because Mylia loves the "Cookie Monster," we adopt the *Sesame Street* theme, complete with tablecloth, favors, etc.. We find an educational action toy that makes *Sesame Street* sounds. When Mac arrives with a huge balloon and the camera, the party begins. Mylia "hams" the entire time. Mac takes loads of pictures, which after filling up two pages in our family photo album, we share with Miss Lacy and the foster mom. With children like Mylia, time is the enemy; it is best not to defer some events for the future but to facilitate and capture special moments in time. Mylia's third birthday is wonderful!

Another great memory occurs when her class has a field trip to "Chuck-E-Cheese" The eatery that we visit is located in Towson, Maryland on Goucher Boulevard. It features a huge area for duck-pin bowling, a large area for the consumption of pizza and other foods, and a game area.

I am enthusiastic about this outing because Mylia has missed most of the others due to illness, clinic appointments, etc. Enroute, I wonder what will be done to accommodate the children's wheelchairs. Not to worry —a gadget is placed at each approach that holds the ball and controls its direction. At first, Mylia can not grasp the concept of "taking turns" to bowl, but after a few tears and a half hearted attempt to launch a temper tantrum, she grasps the concept, participates with gusto, and ends up with the highest average on her team. Her little face, wreathed in smiles, attests to the fun she has while riding on the helicopter.

At about this time I realize that her current foster parents are coping, and apparently plan to keep her. As with times before, I do battle with myself. My rational self realizes that stability is very important in Mylia's case; she has been moved too many times already. My other self focuses on the better quality of life that we are able to give her. The battle lasts for a brief time, and then the rational self wins.

JEANNE C. WHITE

Chapter 5

Working Our Way through the System

I continue to see Mylia and share in her life on the days I spend at Barton, and I keep Mac abreast of what is happening. He wants to be her "daddy," but realizes, with each day that she spends with her current foster parents, the less the likelihood that we'll ever have her. One day, like a bolt from out of the blue, the idea occurs to us, almost simultaneously, that, what we are willing to do for Mylia, we can do for another little girl with the same medical problems.

We decide that we will seek a little girl, 18 months of age, give or take several months. We want an Afro-American, who is HIV positive, possibly a child who is an orphan or who has been abandoned. The age and race are factors because of the "bonding" issue, and gender matters because of our "track" records with girls. We dare to seek just one child, but if the situation arises in which sibling are involved, we will accept more than one. Our sole mission at this point is to "rescue the perishing."

Next, we decide on the child welfare organization that has the best record for placements, support services, etc. I try to contact Mylia's social worker, but she never returns my calls, and as a consequence, I question her commitment to children, including Mylia. It is a fact that workers are often overloaded and under paid, but this worker's inability to find time to return my call makes me wonder how affective her agency is in placing children, transitioning them, and in supporting foster parents.

Eventually, my quest results in a referral to Angel Charities, and we decide to make contact.

Upon our very first meeting with the training director, we are convinced that we have come to the best source. Ms. Berman, as she will be called, doesn't have that "dowdy" look characteristic of many social workers. She suggests rather, a cover model for a magazine for large boned women. Her ash blond hair in a short no nonsense cut, is peppered with grey, but her face holds vestiges of youth. Her chic business like attire, her innate dignity, and the aplomb with which she fields our barrage of questions, dispel any anxieties.

Under her direction, we begin training—thirty hours of informative meetings with other prospective foster parents, and staff members. We learn how the "system" works, the nature of children in foster care, characteristics of "birth" mothers, how to avoid/handle allegations of abuse, etc. We spend a Saturday in C.P.A. training. Our training contains very little information related to the specific child whom we seek. Sometimes I am bored; my background in education and child psychology has included much of the information. So much attention is focused on the emotionally disturbed child and the nonsocial behaviors of many of the children in foster care, that if we are not truly committed, we will have second thoughts. We discuss, in private, if the scary focus on children who lie, steal, set fires, act out sexually, isn't just a ploy to deter anyone who is not truly committed.

We hang in faithfully, <u>knowing</u> that we can cope with a medically fragile child, <u>sure</u> that we can fill her life with happiness and love. We complete the extensive paperwork on time, paperwork that includes a lengthy autobiography. In addition to the forms, there are criminal background checks, driving record checks, physical examinations, home checks by the training director, health, and fire departments, and requests for letters of reference.

As our training proceeds uneventfully, our anticipation grows.

To quell it, we engage a "used" furniture dealer to rid our guest room of its contents. It feels great to take a last look at the old Spanish provincial furniture. My Afro-American doll collection is given a new space in the den. Next we spruce up the walls, and begin the "fun" part—readying the room for a little one. At Hechinger's, we find enough borders with brown and pink bears to cover the top and middle of the walls. Next, we purchase an ornate crib with drop sides, that because of its size, will serve a young child quite well. We make up the bed with a pink and green comforter, pink sheets, a pink bumper, and a white teddy bear for added effect. On this day, we also set in place, a white dresser/bureau and a little white chair, guaranteed for safety by *Good Housekeeping*.

On the next shopping spree, we secure a yellow playpen, a Graco stroller, a car seat that we have investigated via *Consumer's Guide*, a high chair and a "potty chair." Now, a child must have toys and books, so our next excursion results in an assortment of these.

Throughout this time of training and preparation, I continue to spend many days at the Barton School in close contact with Mylia. Being with her brings much happiness and satisfaction, and enables me to contain my excitement about the child we expect. Mylia has blossomed in Miss Lacy's class. She has learned her name, and she calls her teacher "Lacy" instead of "Ma." She knows and understands many words, talks in short sentences, and counts from one to five. Most impressive is that she feels secure enough to trade her bottle for a cup.

Mac and I are optimistic as we near the end of our training for there have been no snags. We think that a child will be placed with us because most foster parents, mainly because of fear, do not actively seek HIV positive children. Training lasts from January through the first week in April. April comes and goes; May comes and goes, and we have no child. The training director feels us out on whether we will consider an older boy. In a testy manner, I remind her that our position has been clear from the beginning in terms of age, gender, and needs. At this point, Mac is peeved also, but he is better at concealing his feelings than I am. We suspect that someone is "playing games" or "playing God," only not with us, but with an Afro-American child for whom the time may be running out. Since both of us are sensitive to the Afro-American's plight, past and present, we wonder if a child of any other race will, with the availability of a home, have to wait. Both of us realize, from my experience with Mylia, that the warm months bode well for HIV children in terms of fewer colds, infections, etc.

As is her custom, the training director tries to placate us in her cool, calm way, but we do not internalize her excuses. All that we know is that a little girl might miss her last chance for summer fun because of "red tape." We submit that if Angel Charities as an agency, cannot access the system to find a child for us, then perhaps we need to try to access it on our own. Since the source of children in foster care is D.S.S., can the smaller agencies work together for the sake of a child?

Immediately, I embark on my mission to access the "system." I jot down names and phone numbers of the administrators at the Department of Social Services, H.E.R.O., The Kennedy-Kreiger Center, B.A.R.C. etc., I clip ads seeking homes for foster children from weekly and daily papers, highlighting all of them that place HIV positive children. The training director realizes that I am serious in my intention to access the system. Just when I have my strategy mapped out, she informs us that her agency is now actively in search of a child for us.

June arrives, and we are still waiting. I step up my efforts starting first with the statewide coordinator. He hears me out and apologetically refers me to some one who might be more helpful. In all, I talk with a total of five persons, all of whom are polite and interested, but unable to say with certainty where a child waits. One administrator tries to interest me in his agency, but I inform him that we have no intention of going through another licensing process. He promises that if his agency receives a child like the one we seek, he will contact us. If we wish to proceed with his agency, we can sign a waiver to have our records forwarded from Angel Charities.

June 5th comes and goes, and I am on another emotional "roller coaster," experiencing a gamut of conflicting emotions—exasperation with the administrators of Angel Charities for not finding a child for us yet, but satisfaction that they are now, at least, trying; sadness that a little girl is missing out on a lot, but happiness, that for one more day, we are free to come and go at will.

JEANNE C. WHITE

Chapter 6

Rays of Hope

Friday, June 17th arrives, and at 6 a.m., the day promises to be oppressively hot. It will be another "code red day," which means that the combination of heat and humidity will cause problems for the very young, the elderly, and those with respiratory conditions. We make plans to remain in the comfort of our air conditioned home during the day and visit the lake area in Columbia, Maryland later in the evening. About 9 a.m., the phone rings. The caller is Isaac, one of the staff members at the agency. He wants us to know that he is aware of our frustrations with "the system" that we had articulated so clearly the previous evening at the "Support Group" session (designed for those awaiting a child). He also wants to inform us that a child has been matched with us. HALLELUJAH!!! For a moment, we are jubilant, but then "caution" rears its head, and common sense prevails. Other foster parents have told us of how they had been matched with a child, only to have "the deal fall through at the last moment. We decide on the "seeing is believing" approach.

Two hours later, Betty, the social worker who has been assigned to us, calls to echo Isaac's news. She gives the child's name, which is Marie, and reminds us that we have already met her when we visited the group home at the end of the training. Betty says that she will schedule an appointment for the following week so that she can familiarize us with Marie's medical history.

Now, we do have a ray of hope, because we realize that we have interacted with Marie, not only once, but twice.

We first meet Marie in April 1994 as the very last part of our training. We visit a group home that houses HIV positive infants and toddlers. Of the seven little ones in residence at that time, we are drawn to Marie because she is the shyest of the group, and the "picture of health" despite her diagnosis. Marie is short and plump, balanced well on sturdy legs. Her impish face is framed by a thick suit of hair that is tightly plaited in corn rows. Mac knows how I detest this style that dates back to slavery, so he anticipates my message when I whisper that "I wish I could get Marie just for a day. I would make changes in her hair a priority." Marie is dressed neatly in sportswear and Keds, but the outfit is too roomy. I sneak a peek when she inches close to us and discover the reason. It is a "T4." My huge earrings fascinate her so much that I am able to sit her on my lap. When I sing and pantomime "Ten Little Indians," she glows. We stay a while longer, enjoying ourselves immensely. As we leave, the director of the home asks us if we would consider taking a child older than the eighteen months we had mentioned. Mac and I assure her of the possibility, especially if it means that we can have Marie.

We meet Marie for the second time at the annual picnic held in June for the families, friends, etc., with ties to the group home. She remembers "Ten Little Indians" which I sing twice. We each hold her during the picnic.

The day we get good news from both Isaac and Betty that we will get Marie is a day worth remembering. It marks the sixth month since we have been involved in our quest to rescue a child. The anxiety and frustration give way to inner peace and optimism, and we can hardly wait for the appointment with Betty the following week.

Tuesday, June 21st dawns hot and muggy, but we are oblivious to the elements as we arrive for the appointment with Betty. In fact, we arrive thirty-five minutes early. Once it starts,

Betty handles the proceedings with ease, thoughtfully leaving Mac and me alone to read Marie's medical history.

This child, like Mylia, must have a strong will to survive, for the neglect, deprivation, and multiple health problems that she has experienced, almost parallel those experienced by Mylia. Marie's health is much improved because of the excellent care she has received at the group home. As we read and comment, Mac and I vow that we will not be the ones to fail this child. We just hope that "the system" works to transition her smoothly and quickly because every minute counts. We discover that we have just missed her second birthday, but we hope that with love, laughter, and excellent care, she will live to enjoy a huge party when she reaches three—our promise.

Betty sets up a meeting with the staff of the group home for transitioning Marie from the group home to ours. With great excitement and expectation, we listen and take notes. To our delight, Marie is brought in. She recognizes us instantly and climbs up on my lap. A second later, she moves into Mac's arms. There will be no problems with bonding. After a short visit, Marie is removed, to her obvious dismay. As the team finalizes the schedule, Marie peeps at us through the French doors and plays "peek-a boo."

The intense transitioning will cover three weeks, progressing from "in-house" visits to "home-day-visits" to "home-overnight-visits." All of this, in our opinion, seems a bit much. But we'll do it. It will be August before Marie is ours, and many of our planned activities will have to be cancelled.

The "in house" meetings with Marie go well. She is so bright, and her mind is a "sponge." She repeats three and four syllable words, and expresses herself in sentences. We assist in her mealtime and bath-time rituals with mutual enjoyment.

Events are moving along so smoothly that we breath easier, trying to believe that "the system" will not fail Marie nor us. Even when I fracture my ankle in a freak accident, we persevere with the schedule, determined to arm no one with a reason to alter the course. For Marie's first "home-day-visit," we plan to take her to the annual steelworkers' picnic. The day arrives, a Sunday, and we call for Marie at 10 a.m. Her caretaker has dressed her in a sleeveless dress, white socks edged in tiny blue bows, and Nike shoes. Her hair has been oiled and styled in four twists. She looks adorable, but she is not dressed for a picnic. We have anticipated this situation and have bought her a one piece playsuit, color coordinated with blue and white accessories. As soon as we reach the site of the picnic, I change her clothes. The 24 month size outfit, although a little baggy, is a good fit.

What a wonderful day! The heat is stifling under a glaring sun, but the century old trees and foliage in Patapsco State Park, serve as a buffer and make an ideal place for the picnic. Marie is relaxed with us in this unfamiliar setting, and is eager to learn the names of all objects. She won't let Mac out of her sight. He is the "ticket taker" for the day, and his post is nearby. Whenever Marie cannot make eye contact with him, she calls "Pop-Pop" and he comes immediately, much to her delight. I take Marie for a walk and she says, "Hi" to everyone. During the day, I keep on schedule with Marie's snacks, meals, and medication. Of the snacks that I have packed, she loves the pared apple slices best. Of the picnic menu, she likes the baked beans.

We have brought along the stroller, and although I have doubts that she will go to sleep, I position her. Miracles of miracles! Marie takes a nap, and she does so in spite of loud music, voices, etc. When she awakens, the first thing she does is to look for and call "Pop-Pop." She plays ball with some of the children, and I catch many pictures on film. Marie "hams" before the camera, as usual.

An approaching thunderstorm causes us to run to the pavilion. The rain is warm, and I hold Marie's little hands outside of the pavilion so that she can feel it. I say "rain," and she repeats the word while rubbing the moisture on her cheeks. Snap! Mac has captured this on film. Marie is due back at the home at

4 p.m. Thus, as soon as the storm ends, I change her and feed her, and we leave the park. Lord, it's been a mighty good day!

Several days after the picnic, a day begins and ends with "Trouble," spelled with a capital T. The day echoes the proverbial belief that trouble "comes in threes." First, we are wakened ,at 3 a.m. with the restless stirring of our doberman, Majesty. Mac rises to let him out into the "run" and discovers, through his nose, that Majesty has "pooped" in the living room. Now this is most unusual for Majesty, and we connect immediately with the cause. Majesty has just spent the previous day with the vet having his teeth cleaned. We should have remembered that he gets diarrhea each time that he is anesthetized. Mac cleans up and shampoos the section of the carpet before returning to bed.

The next event occurs at 9 a.m. of the same day. Betty calls to share some news with both of us. "Bad news" we mouth to each other as we position ourselves. "I have a little bad news," Betty says. "It seems that now there is a glitch in the plan to discharge Marie on the last Thursday in July. Someone has not filed certain papers regarding funding, and as a result, the scheduled date of discharge has been changed." Betty says, "Don't worry!" Her advice falls on deaf ears as I am close to tears, and Mac's face is now cast with an ash-like pallor.

We should have braced ourselves. Things have been going too smoothly. This is like a sadistic game played with human emotions. We love and want Marie, and she loves us. How can "the system" that hires so many people and expects so much of its foster parents, fall so short in its operational practices?

How can those who control the destinies of thousands of children fail to understand the pain and heartache that result from incomplete or haphazard paperwork? We vent our pain; we understand why many well-intentioned foster and/or adoptive parents drop out of training and change their minds. For one moment, we consider saying 'To hell with it" and going back to our original plans for retirement. But we remember Mylia, who is the catalyst for our actions, and we see Marie's face and hear her saying "Okey-Dokey," and we realize that we've come too far, spent too much money, invested all of our love, and we won't give up.

Thoughts of "giving up" surface momentarily again when "trouble" pops up for the third time in one day with a call from Mac's urologist. Prior to beginning our training as foster parents, Mac had from time to time experienced discomfort in his abdomen and side. All previous tests had come up negative, but on this day his doctor calls with unsettling news. The most recent test has indicated a cause for his discomfort, and the doctor wants Mac to come to his office right away. On a day that, up to this point has been draining, a new threat looms and ushers in a cloud of gloom. I accompany Mac, and the doctor says that Mac must have prompt major surgery for "colo-vesicle fistula."

As we leave, we are stunned into silence, knowing that we have to talk, but unable to do so now. Neither of us sleeps well that night as we ponder personal coping strategies, and to what degree the surgery will impact upon Marie's transitioning. The following morning, we sort through our fears and anxieties. We debate putting the transitioning on hold. We decide to proceed because according to Betty, the date of discharge is in question. Mac wonders if I can handle Marie's overnight visits without him. I assure him that I can manage, but I admit it will be hard, if not impossible, to be a presence and a comfort through the surgery with a two year old in tow. The only solution is to share our information with Betty and the staff of the group home, affirm our intention to continue with the transitioning, but ask for a few modifications. After all, we have cooperated with them and adapted our lives with sincerity to their expectations. Is it too much to ask that they modify the schedule for us? It has been a "hell" of a 24 hours.

Mac's surgery is scheduled for Tuesday, August 9th. We put thoughts of it back in our minds so that we can enjoy Marie.

We take her to church one Sunday, and she acts as pretty as she looks in the outfit we have purchased just for this occasion.

I take her for walks around the neighborhood to familiarize her with it. We go to Security Mall and she is mesmerized by the fountain. She wants to toss in more pennies than we have, so we have to divert her attention. Mac takes her to Woodlawn cemetery to feed the swans. She isn't afraid of them even when they approach her. We visit the library for "story time," and we borrow three books for her to enjoy at naptime.

Betty calls on July 28th to give us an update. It seems the funding issue has been settled, but now there is a holdup with the paperwork. Betty is going on vacation, and she hopes to have good news when she returns. As for us, we are managing to hold on to one little ray of hope, that in due time Marie will come to stay.

JEANNE C. WHITE

Chapter 7

Time To Rejoice

August 1st comes and goes with no word from Betty on Marie's discharge date. I am extremely anxious about Mac's upcoming surgery, which is scheduled for August 9th. He avoids the subject as a way of dealing with his own anxieties, and this leaves me wrestling silently with all manner of thoughts. After all, the very nature of the surgery and the four hour duration as predicted by his doctor, suggest an event of no minor significance. It is Marie who enables me to keep things in perspective. As we continue to have her for overnight visits, I focus on the reality of her needs at the moment as opposed to dwelling on the "unknowns" of the outcome of the surgery.

It is thoughts of Marie that propel me through my long solitary vigil at the hospital on the 9th. I trust that the power of Mac's love for me, and for her will give him the will to bear the surgery and recuperate from it. That same night, Betty calls and boosts my spirits by notifying me of Marie's discharge date, August 18th. Oh! What I wouldn't give to be able to share this news with Mac! Past experiences with "the system" flood my mind, and I am determined to "bridle my tongue" just in case.

The surgery is a success, and Mac's doctor foresees no complications. I am uplifted on my daily visits to see Mac improving steadily. He wants to know about Marie and how she is responding to his absence. Since I have continued on with the "transitioning" schedule, I can honestly relate that Marie misses him greatly. Even though we do many "fun" things, she keeps asking "Where is Pop-pop"? The hospital's visitation policy allows visits by children. I promise both him and her that I will bring her to see "Pop-pop" just as soon as he is up to it. The day of our visit proves to be a mutual "treat." Mac's face lights up so much that for a second I am a bit jealous. Marie seems a bit puzzled that "Pop-pop" doesn't pick her up as usual, but she does flips, jabbers, sings, etc., and just basks in the attention she gets from him. Some experts believe that very young children cannot comprehend abstracts such as illness, death, etc, but I believe that Marie can because she doesn't ever again ask, "Where is Pop-pop?" She just seems to know and to be at peace with the knowledge.

As usual, the course of Marie's discharge is not a smooth one. The date, August 18th, remains the same, but the actual time is changed three times. Marie is on a "home visit" for the two days and nights prior to the 18th. Originally, I had made plans to dress Marie up special for the occasion, but with so many changes in time, I begin to doubt that the discharge will occur. Consequently, when I take her back to the home, she is dressed in a faded blue and white dress that she has brought with her. I do make two concessions—instead of returning her clothes in the plastic bag with which she has come, I pack her belongings in Samsonite luggage; I also put new "Mermaid" sneakers on her little feet.

Glory Hallelujah! When we arrive at the group home, a little early at 12:45 p.m., Betty and a social worker from D.S.S. are already there. My heart almost jumps out of my body! It is really going to happen! At last! A child—not the little one Mylia, who got us started on this path, but one just as dear and just as much in need, Marie—will have a home! By 2 p.m. the paperwork is complete. Marie and I set off for the hospital to share the joyous news with Mac. There we get more good news. He is going to be discharged the following day.

Nothing can rob us of the joy that we feel. Not even that

there are no banners, balloons, and family members etc., to celebrate her coming Not even that there are no gooey desserts, sheet cake with Barney figures, and globs of melting ice cream. There will be time for all of this, time for much more than this. All that matters right now is that our mission has been accomplished; we have rescued one child.

Later when Mac has recovered from surgery, and when my ankle has healed, we can have the formal celebration. Today we rejoice in the presence of this little one and in the opportunity to shower her with the love that she needs and deserves. We rejoice in the opportunity to provide her with the best care possible. We rejoice that Marie has a home of her own.

J E A N N E C. W H I T E

Chapter 8

Daily Life with Our Child

Life with a two-year-old is full of both fun and challenges. We have embraced this life with confidence due to in part to the very structured nature of my essence. Marie's day begins at 6:00 a.m. when she is roused for a Pamper change and her dosage of several medications. Sometimes she goes right back to sleep, which gives me the luxury of an uninterrupted bath, and Mac an extra few minutes of sleep. Sometimes, instead of returning to sleep, she jumps up and down in her crib and calls "Mom-Mom" or "Pop- Pop" every two seconds. At 7:00 a.m. I get her up and prepare her for the day. She gets a lotion massage which she loves because she gets to smear gobs of lotion on both of us. By 8:00 a.m., she has enjoyed a hearty breakfast, had her hair combed, and is ready for a walk.

We watch squirrels scamper across lawns, and we sing songs, and play games such as "red light—green light" to practice following directions. Because Marie is visibly frightened by loud noises, I have her name airplanes, lawn-mowers, etc. and wave at busses, cars, trucks, etc. Her little eyes light up when drivers honk their horns and wave to her. The elementary and middle school students, enroute to the neighborhood schools respond to her friendliness with waves and greetings. The traffic guard at the corner of our block actually looks for her everyday.

After our walk, there is "circle time" until 10:00 a.m. Mac, Marie, one of our dogs, Kermit, rabbit (stuffed toys), and I join in this "guided play" time with shapes, colors, numbers, and art work. Following a snack of milk and cheese or fruit at 10 a.m., we sing songs and enjoy stories. The songs usually entail actions and include "The Farmer in the Dell" and "Old MacDonald." For one half hour before lunch, Marie plays independently. HER TOYS ARE EVERYWHERE! During this period, we can expect her to come to either of us with a "real" or "imaginary" boo-boo. If a kiss is not enough, she'll ask for "ice" to put on it or a "tissue to wipe the tears." This little one is a "born ham."

Noon ushers in lunch and medicine. I prepare a well balanced hot meal which Marie eats with "gusto." At times, she crams food into her mouth, but with a gentle reminder from us, along with a few guided spoons, she proceeds slowly again.

Nap time follows lunch and lasts until 2:30 or 3:00 p.m. I use this time to do the daily laundry, read the newspaper, work crossword puzzles, etc. Marie gets a light snack when she awakens from her nap. While I prepare dinner, Mac engages her in games such as "Tag" or "Follow the Leader," games that involve much movement and body coordination.

We eat dinner at 5:00 p.m. after which Marie gets to go for a walk, ride her tricycle, blow bubbles, or engage in some other type of outdoor activity. Just before her bath at 6:00 p.m., I give Marie her medicines. We have a variety of bathtub toys, but bubbles seems to capture her attention most of the time. She gets her last snack at 7:15 p.m., and then the three of us snuggle on the sofa in the den and watch video. At 8:00 p.m., Marie says her prayers, gets kisses and hugs, and generally goes immediately to sleep. The day ends at midnight when Mac gives her last medicines for the day and changes her pamper.

Marie's schedule is flexible by necessity, because of "potty training," clinic appointments, visits with her social worker, etc. Yet, having a schedule in place enables us to provide her with a variety of quality experiences. If an opportunity arises for her to play with other toddlers, we "go for it." We honestly admit to ourselves that she learns more about sharing and "taking turns" from her peers.

Fridays are usually reserved for field trips, but if an event for children falls on another day, we secure tickets and attend. We go to the market and to the mall on Saturdays. We marvel at how an ordinary activity such as buying groceries becomes an adventure when it is being done with a toddler. Sundays are spent attending church and interacting with our families. Marie knows when Sunday arrives because of the aromas that emanate from the kitchen.

Life with Marie is so rewarding. Daily we can see the results of our efforts. Her skin is clearer; her hair is less dry; she is gaining weight; most of all, she has confidence that we love her unconditionally and will keep her safe. This faith humbles us before God and man.

J E A N N E C. W H I T E

Chapter 9

Blest Be the Tie That Binds

It is September with a typical pattern of warm days and chilly nights. We are enjoying Marie so much, and in preparation for Halloween, have purchased a bunny costume. Our "circle times" include making masks from paper bags, coloring and cutting out pumpkins, and stories about Halloween. Not a day passes that I don't think and talk about Mylia, and with the opening of school, I know that through Ms. Lacy, I can keep abreast of her activities. I give Ms. Lacy a few days to get back into the swing of things before I call her. She says Mylia has not returned from summer vacation. When I follow up on this news with a call to her foster mom, I learn that Mylia has just been released from the hospital because of an infection, and is being visited daily by a nurse. This news is quite distressing despite the assurances of her foster mom that Mylia is getting better. I recall just before school closed in June, Mylia was refusing to eat and losing weight. I believe that during the summer, without the joy, laughter, and love from her friends in the school, she has lost her reason to fight. One week later, the phone rings at 10:30 p.m. . It is one of my friends at school calling to alert me that Mylia is again in the hospital and that her condition is critical. Without a moment's hesitation, I call the foster mom, who confirms the news. She says "Mylia has been in the critical care unit since Saturday night, and the medical team has said that her death can come at any time."

I reply, "I intend to visit her tomorrow."

She replies, "Don't expect much."

Overwhelmed with sadness, I do not sleep. To Mac, who also cannot sleep, I verbalize my hope that Mylia will hold on until I get there. By 9:00 a.m. the following morning, Mac, Marie, and I are at Union Hospital. They settle in the lobby, and I secure a pass and head for the pediatric I.C.U.

I think that I am prepared emotionally to handle Mylia's death, but I am not. The sight of her confirms what I have been told. Her emaciated little body is in a semi-fetal position beneath a light blanket. A pamper is situated loosely between her legs.

Several tubes protrude from various parts of her body. An oxygen mask dwarfs her face, and her breathing is labored. My child, my little friend, who has fought so valiantly in the past, has very little left with which to fight. She is non-responsive to touch, sound, etc.. She is lying on her side, but this does not prevent me from seeing the deterioration of her face and the dark, thick substance that oozes from her mouth. I take her cool hands in mine, talk to her, and seek in some way to let her know who I am. I try to sing "The Barney Song" but my lips won't form the words. Instead, my tears flow in torrents.

Until this time, I have not paid attention to any details of the room, but now I spot a number of bags and adult garments. When the bathroom door opens, I discover that I have not been alone in the room. When I introduce myself, I learn that Mylia's "birth" mom and dad are staying with Mylia. Her mom says that the police tracked them down on the day after Mylia was admitted. In another time, the circumstances of this woman's life, might have resulted in a rift between us, but today we are drawn to each other. We are "soul" sisters sharing the pain of losing a child. I tell her of the wonderful times that Mylia had at the school, and I tell her of the birthday party that she had. She shares with me the fact that for she is homeless, but that her social worker is trying to get her in a shelter. She and I end up crying in each other's arms, offering comfort to each other.

I tell her, "Since you brought Mylia into this world, it is altogether good and fitting that you are here at the end." What I do not tell her is that her presence has eliminated a fear that I have harbored for some time—the fear that Mylia would die alone.

I return to stand by Mylia's bed for a while longer. If only I could hold her one more time. I share this with a nurse who comes in, but she tells me, "It is better if Mylia stays as still as possible." My visit lasts about 45 minutes. As I say, "Bye-bye," for what I know is the last time, I need to believe that Mylia held on until I could get to her.

A farewell hug is what I offer to her mother, and then I leave the room. When I return to Mac and report on Mylia's condition, he decides against going to see her. He is the one who answers the phone at 5:30 a.m. the following morning when Mylia's foster mom calls to say, "Mylia died at 4:30 p.m."

Mac is an excellent sounding board, and because he understands the depth of my love for Mylia, I am able to verbalize my feelings and to grieve without shame. Two days after Mylia's death, I talk with Ms. Lacy by phone. She and I wonder if in light of the circumstances there will be a funeral. Ms. Lacy says, "Perhaps Mylia will be cremated," and I SHUDDER AT THE THOUGHT. There is relief when her foster mom calls to say that there will be a funeral on the following Tuesday, almost a week to the day when she died. Now with this news, Mac and I can do what we need to do to add closure. We visit a local florist and decide on a floral tribute that will be small enough to fit in Mylia's casket. Our selection is a satin pillow covered with pink carnations and baby's breath, topped with a pink bow. I write on the card, "We shall love you forever." The pillow's place inside the coffin allows us the way to seal a part of us with her for eternity.

The day of Mylia's funeral is sunny and cool with a brisk wind that prompts us to wear lightweight coats. The director of the group home, upon being informed by me of Mylia's death, and having known Mylia from her days as a resident of the home, extends the invitation for Marie to stay there while we attend the funeral. We accept her invitation and drop Marie off there at 9:45 a.m.. It seems I am toting about 75 extra pounds of sadness and grief. When we arrive at the funeral home, its location in a rundown area of the city does little for my mental state. We spot a few familiar faces among the small assembly— Mylia's mother, father, and sister, her foster parents, and several other staff members from the Barton School and the aide on the bus that Mylia rode. We're sure that there are some social workers in attendance, because from our work with "the system," we have found social workers to be involved in all major life and death events, and because there are some young, business-like women sitting towards the rear of the room.

It seems as if my feet lock in place as we approach the casket, and Mac sort of propels me forward. With blurred vision, I gaze on the face, a face that in the finality of death bears just a slight resemblance to the Mylia that I have known. She is dressed in white, and her thin hair is curled loosely around her face. The pillow of flowers that we ordered is in one corner of the casket. Mac and I sit in the back of Ms. Lacy, in full view of Mylia, and for the entire hour of the service, I observe a vigil for my friend. The thick wad of kleenex in my palm comes in handy as I use it to muffle my sobs.

The musician pumps out loud "heavy" gospel music such as "Going Up Yonder," music totally inappropriate for Mylia. "Jesus Loves Me" or "When He Cometh" would have been better. I tune out the prayers and the eulogy, preferring instead to recall some of the fun times with Mylia. At the end of the service, in compliance with the mortician's directions, we pass Mylia's open casket as we exit the building. We join with the small cortege for the ride to the cemetery, and once there, Mac helps to bear Mylia's casket to the burial site. In the glare of the bright sun, the cheap casket which is smudged and torn in one place, looks mighty forlorn. Mercifully the minister's prayer is short. As we leave, I look back at the unadorned casket and its site, which will probably never have a marker, and I silently lament, that even in death, the little child, who gave so much has been cheated.

My only consolation comes from knowing that I have been loyal to my little friend from the first day that I met her. Being with her as she drew her last breaths, and through her funeral and burial, enables me to bring closure to her existence. Had I not been able to participate in the last rituals, I would have felt guilty of failing her just as almost everyone else has done.

In "A Psalm of Life" by William Wadsworth Longfellow are these words:

> *Not in enjoyment and not in sorrow,*
> *Is our destined end or way,*
> *But to act that each tomorrow*
> *Find us farther than today.*

Because of Mylia and the thousands of children like her, allover the world, whatever time I have left in my life will be spent in acting on behalf of these dear ones. The "Action Plan" that my husband and I have formulated has three parts:

1. We plan to keep Marie (even if it involves legal steps) and provide her with a quality life of love, fun, and security.
2. We plan to act as a "committee of two" to recruit other retired couples like us as parents for children like Mylia.
3. We plan to set up a fund in Mylia's name that will perpetuate her memory and influence on all those who knew her, a fund that will provide funds for field trips, excursions, perhaps even a camp. This last part is by far the most important because we can't delay! Now is the time to do something wonderful for at least some of these little ones in Mylia's memory!

J E A N N E C. W H I T E

The Afterword

The author wishes to explain why this account is written in the present tense. When I began this work, Mylia was alive and I had hope. Even though she died before its completion, I need to keep her alive in my thoughts:

1. To delay facing up to the reality that, for Mylia and others like her, a cure for AIDS will not come in time.
2. To keep me ever aware of what I must do now to keep Mylia and others like her, before the public, to combat ignorance and fear, and to replace these with compassion and love.
3. To generate zeal, money, time, etc. in search of a cure for this illness that affects all races, genders, and ages, including babies.